GONE FOR GOOD!

The End of Yo-Yo Dieting

SUSAN N. LEWIS RN,BSN

ISBN: 1492258652
ISBN 13: 9781492258650
Library of Congress Control Number: 2013915623
CreateSpace Independent Publishing Platform
North Charleston, South Carolina

TABLE OF CONTENTS

INTRODUCTION

Congratulations! You've made it! You've counted, sweated, starved, juiced, detoxed, and done just about anything to lose weight. You've pumped iron, run, cycled, and Zumba'ed up a sweat seven days a week. And it worked! You've met your goal. Now what?

I run a very successful weight-loss program and function as a personal weight-loss coach. I'm not going to bore you with all of the details of those programs, because that's not what this book is about. While I genuinely do believe that I have a superior program to lose those unwanted pounds, I also know that there are many, many ways to lose weight. Some are healthy, and some are not, but they exist, nevertheless.

This is not a weight-loss plan. Hundreds of those already exist. No, I'm writing about a subject that is even closer to my heart: how to keep the weight off once you've lost it. In my practice, I have had hundreds of patients tell me about their many diet attempts. Every patient has told me how much weight has been lost with each diet. If I add up all the weight lost on each program for just one person, it totals hundreds of pounds—hundreds of pounds lost over the course of one person's lifetime! And yet, they all keep gaining it back. And sadly, they gain back more weight than they originally lost. As they recount their stories through their tears, I can see the frustration, despair, and hopelessness in their faces. I can hear it in their voices. My heart is touched, because this is truly a dilemma.

Yo-yo dieting, also known as weight cycling, is a real problem in this country. We lose, we gain. Up, down, repeat. Psychologically and emotionally, this yo-yo effect causes untold counts of depression, fatigue, and low self-esteem. People feel like failures. They are ashamed and embarrassed. They don't want anyone to know that they're weak and lack discipline, so they never share what they're going through.

I also learned from my patients and clients that they—like myself—had totally lost faith in the "system" of dieting. They were tired of trying the latest thing. They realized that the information coming to them through normal media outlets was not accurate or even well intentioned. They came to the conclusion that they were being given information with no other purpose than to make money for the manufacturer or advertiser. The people who came into my office were sick and tired of being lied to and manipulated. They were exhausted with a system that allowed it to happen.

About seven years ago, I set out to find a solution—a simple solution at that. Anyone who has been through my program knows my core belief: food is not the enemy we've made it out to be. I don't believe that we're meant to spend our lives counting calories, grams of fat, or anything else. I don't believe that we must spend three hours in the gym every day to burn off calories so that we won't gain weight.

I believe that life and food are meant to be enjoyed. The food of our ancestors was not complicated. Modern man has made it so. But I believe that we can get back to eating simple, clean, real food that our bodies respond to and recognize. I think that food can be delicious and satisfying. And I don't think it has to be that hard.

I have developed this philosophy over the past seven years. During this time, I have been researching, documenting, and, most of all, listening to and observing my patients. My goal in writing this book is to share the knowledge I have gained through the experiences I have had with these patients. It is truly my privilege and joy to share the results of these experiences with you.

I will not bore you with a lot of research and scientific material. Other books, as well as various Internet sites, are available if you would like to do additional research. I'm here to give you the basics of eight simple keys that will greatly increase your ability to keep the weight off through healthy means. These eight keys are based on the feedback and observations of patients who have been through my program and have kept the weight off. They have given me a clear picture about what doesn't work and what really, really does work.

KEY ONE: DON'T SKIMP ON PROTEIN

Twenty-five to forty percent of food intake should be lean protein. The word here is *lean*. Bacon, salami, and deli meat do not count. Our ancestors hunted and fished for their food. Game, fish, and other marine mammals were the most abundant food source around. Other food sources—like berries, fruits, nuts, and greens (which were really wild grasses)—existed but were much less available, depending on the geographical region and the weather. They were also much harder and time-consuming to collect. The vegetables and other agricultural products we eat today did not even exist. Grains and cereals that are so prevalent in our diet today did not exist. Evidence shows that we still have the genetic make-up of our ancestors, and as such, we do not easily tolerate these agriculturally grown or processed foods. Our bodies really don't even know how to handle or digest some of these foods.

Our bodies are composed mainly of proteins. Proteins provide the building blocks needed to replace worn or damaged cells. Proteins from animal sources are considered a complete protein since they contain all nine of the essential amino acids. Vegetable proteins are incomplete because they lack at least one of the essential amino acids and must be combined with other amino acids to become complete. In this book, my reference to protein means *animal* protein.

Even so, it has become very popular to dismiss and criticize eating any animal proteins. These critics maintain that plant-based diets are best for our bodies, as well as our planet. There are several problems with these arguments.

First, it is impossible to get the right proteins into our bodies if we eat only fruits and vegetables. The proponents of these diets state that it is possible to combine the right vegetables and starches (grains) to form a complete protein. Technically this is true. This explains why sending rice and beans to poor countries allows the inhabitants of those countries to stave off protein depravation. But this is a poor substitute for real protein.

Additionally, combining foods correctly in order to provide these nine essential proteins to our bodies is not only time-consuming but also requires a certain amount of education and understanding about these proteins and the amino-acid chains that comprise them. For example, in the above mentioned beans-and-rice explanation, both of these foods are starchy and will convert easily to sugar, which may contribute to weight gain. That's OK if you're actually starving but usually not OK in our Western world.

There are so many sources of lean protein that most people find it easy to come up with a list of foods that works for them. For example, I don't really like beef, but I really like fish and shrimp. You don't have to include every food in your diet, but branching out and trying something different can be fun and educational. Instead of chicken, have Cornish hen for a change.

Protein is the most important food group for managing blood sugar and reducing the potential for developing diseases like diabetes, high blood pressure, and other health problems. It is interesting to note that, when we study our ancestors, we find that they usually did not show the same signs of osteoporosis, atherosclerosis, or cancer that we currently see in our society. While most of our ancestors died early, their deaths were usually attributed to an accident or war. Anthropologists and archeologists note that, when they examine the remains of a sixty-year old, for example, they find much less of the debilitating health problems that haunt us today. By examining our ancestors, we conclude that some of our current aging and health problems could be a direct result of our poor eating habits. And we know that our ancestors ate large amounts of protein.

EXAMPLES OF LEAN PROTEIN

You may find that many definitions of lean exist. My definition is simple: no overly fatty meats, such as bacon or cuts of meat with obvious amounts of fat. I'm not caught up in beef versus lamb versus pork. Also, beef must be grass fed and organic. This would imply that the product is hormone and antibiotic free. All other products must be naturally raised (usually grass fed or free range) and hormone- and antibiotic-free.

BEEF

Any cut of beef that is grass fed and organic is allowed. Research shows that cows raised in their natural habitat and fed their natural diet do not pack on the same type of saturated fats that are seen in cows raised in commercial feedlots and fed grain. As noted above, grass fed should also mean that there are no antibiotics or hormones in the product. Note that some animal farmers claim that their cows are grass fed, but, in reality, the cows have spent the last twenty or thirty percent of their life eating grain to fatten them up. While this is an improvement over traditional feedlot-raised cows, it still isn't the most ideal. Ask your butcher to be sure.

Lean veal is also allowed.

Eat these no more than two times a month: prime rib, T-bone, rib eye, ribs, and any ground beef over 15 percent fat.

FISH

Any fish is allowed, even fatty fish. However, wild fish is preferred because the type of fat found in wild fish is omega-3, and the type of fat in farm raised is omega-6. In the United States, we get way too much omega-6 and not enough omega-3. This is one of the reasons why I recommend wild fish. Just like cows, fish that are farm raised are usually fed products inconsistent with their natural diet. This explains the difference in types of fat.

Eat these no more than two times a month: tuna, shark, or swordfish.

These large fish are often found to have high levels of mercury and other toxins.

POULTRY

Poultry should be free-range. This means that the animal's entire life has been spent this way, not just a small portion. Again, ask your butcher.

- ✧ Chicken breast
- ✧ Chicken quarter
- ✧ Turkey breast
- ✧ Turkey quarter
- ✧ Cornish hen
- ✧ Duck

EGGS

Purchase omega-3–enriched eggs if possible.

Healthy people do not need to limit their intake of whole eggs. If you have health concerns, such as cholesterol, follow your doctor's advice. Research has shown that, even in folks with high cholesterol, it's safe to eat four to six whole eggs a week. Eliminating the yolk cuts out the fat and cholesterol, and many people choose to eat egg whites only. Note that, contrary to the notion of bodybuilders who eat large amounts of egg whites, the protein content of eggs is less than that of beef or chicken.

LAMB

Lamb has a little less protein and more fat than beef. However, if the lamb is grass fed and hormone-free, then any cut of lamb is allowed. Make sure all cuts are closely trimmed of fat.

PORK

Pork should be raised without hormones or antibiotics. Be sure to cook it well. Pork tenderloin, pork roast, and lean chops are the best choices.

Eat the following no more than two times a month:

    ✧ Bacon
    ✧ Sausage
    ✧ Ham
    ✧ Salami and other preserved meats
    ✧ Deli chicken, turkey, ham, etc.

Better yet, eliminate them altogether. They are treats, not staples.

DAIRY

This is one of the most controversial categories to discuss. Many claim that our ancestors did not drink milk and that we, as humans, have not adapted to having milk products in our bodies. If one buys into the idea that we are at our healthiest when we eat like our ancestors, then this is a true statement.

However, many cultures use large amounts of dairy and dairy fat in their diet and do not have the same health issues that we have in the United States. France is a good example of this. Nowhere are there more dairy products than in France. Butter, cream, and cheese are kitchen staples in just about every region. Again, I suggest that we look at how the animal—whether cow, goat or sheep—is raised. Most animals in France, especially the areas around Provence, are still raised in a pasture, where they eat their natural diet. The fat seen in the milk of these animals is different than the fat seen in the milk of animals raised in a feedlot and fed an unnatural diet of grains.

So what is the best thing to do if you like cream in your coffee? You should:

- Buy only organic.
- Use fat-free products whenever possible, at least in the United States.
- Eat goat cheese; it's easier for most people to digest.
- Buy cheese imported from France (or other areas of Europe) or small dairies (the quality is superior).
- Limit high-fat cheeses, such as Brie.

Try to use dairy as an enhancer—two ounces of skim milk in your coffee, one ounce of hard cheese grated on your salad—or as your dessert. Drinking large quantities of milk may not be in your best interest. Do you really need two large lattes every day?

If you enjoy having cheese before dinner (the American way) or after dinner (the French way), remember to have small servings. When madame serves cheese after dinner, which is a custom always found in a typical French home, she usually brings out a big tray with many selections. However, each person will choose only a very small sliver of two or three cheeses from the selection. If you select a soft cheese, such as Brie, which is best eaten with crackers or bread, limit the crackers or small baguette pieces to no more than two. Otherwise, eat the cheese by itself. You will find it surprisingly flavorful and satisfying if not accompanied by a lot of starchy carbs.

JULIE'S STORY

At the age of sixty-two, Julie realized that something was wrong. The diet and foods that she really thought were healthy were, in fact, contributing to her weight gain, high blood pressure, and borderline diabetes. For seventeen years she was mostly a vegetarian. At least, she ate what she thought a vegetarian should eat. She ate grains—a lot of grains-because she believed that whole grains were healthy and didn't need to be limited. She ate a lot of fruit because it had lots of vitamins and certainly she needed that. She ate lots of beans, carrots, and other highly glycemic vegetables. Occasionally she ate spinach, broccoli and eggs. And over this seventeen-year period, she gained thirty-eight pounds and could not lose it. Nothing worked. Going through menopause made it worse, but she knew that that was not the true problem.

She decided to join a group weight-loss program that she had heard a lot about. She also had a couple of friends who had been on this program in the past and had lost weight. She did well on the program and lost twenty-two pounds in six months, but still did not know how to eat. She ate the foods that they required for their program, but that did not help her in the real world. When she returned to her previous so-called healthy eating style with her *healthy* foods, she started to gain the weight back immediately! She was really discouraged.

She decided to have a free consultation with me to see what different solutions I might offer. At this point, she had no hope of ever keeping the weight off or wearing her size-eight jeans again. But, after doing a short program (six weeks, to be exact), she lost the extra weight and actually learned about food. This was a real eye-opener for her. By using a few really simple rules, she has kept the weight off for four years and with very little effort. When I saw her recently, she was thrilled that her weight was stable *and* that her size-eight jeans looked great! She realized that her body was really craving protein and that she was giving it too many carbohydrates. Even though some of the carbs were OK, she was to-tally out of balance. By adding chicken, fish, and eggs, she feels healthier and looks better. She can even develop muscles when she work out at the gym. She was very grateful that I was able to educate her on proper nutrition for optimal weight maintenance.

KEY TWO: EAT REAL FOOD

A friend of mine, French by birth, once told me that "Americans are so used to eating fake food, they don't know what real food tastes like!" A walk through any US grocery store will confirm my friend's statement. Every package has anywhere from three to thirty ingredients in it. Why?

US food companies know that if they can enhance a product in a certain way, it will encourage, if not downright force, you to eat more of that product. This adds up to a greater profit for the company, though at the expense of your health. Companies add salt, sugar, unhealthy fats, and more chemicals than you can ever imagine. Most Americans don't know that all of these chemicals even exist. If they do read the labels, they assume that all additives are safe, because surely the FDA would not allow anything in our food supply that would harm us. Without getting political, I'm going to strongly suggest that this assumption is incorrect and that not all additives are sufficiently tested (if tested at all) to determine the effects on humans.

Even if a product has been tested for safety, it only suggests that this product is safe by itself. No testing is ever done to determine the health effects of exposure to several chemicals at one time. Since most of our foods have numerous additives—and mostly chemical additives at that—product testing falls well short of convincing us that a food containing all of those chemicals is safe for consumption.

Studies show that ingesting these additives over a period of time is unhealthy for many reasons. Evidence exists that our bodies don't quite recognize chemicals. The liver, which is charged with metabolizing most of these foreign invaders, often has no idea what to do or how to metabolize these chemicals and flush them out of the body. So the liver often chooses to store these toxins in our fat. And, of course, we then need fat to store the toxins. The short version is that this whole process of consuming foreign, made-up products wrecks havoc on our bodies. We gain weight and develop diabetes, high blood pressure, and heart disease.

If you currently eat most of your foods from a package, this will be a challenge for you. To keep weight off and continue a healthy lifestyle, you must consume *real* food, not the stuff that only passes for food.

What do I mean by real food? There are a few rules that will clarify exactly what comprises real food. While the rules are simple, they may take some getting used to. Don't get discouraged. If you have an open mind and really desire to educate yourself, you will be able to conquer this step with relative ease. Most people are able to make this switch within about two weeks.

LIMIT PACKAGED FOODS

Most foods that are sold in some sort of package are really a processed food product. The food has been prepared in some way and has had many ingredients added. If a product has been altered, it is no longer *real*. Peanut butter may not be a real food, unless you grind the nuts yourself or unless the only ingredient on the label is peanuts. Prepared deli turkey breast is not real turkey. Premixed boxes of rice or pasta products are not real—they have too many chemical additives to be recognized by the body as food. Most spice/seasoning blends are not real either. They mostly contain flavor enhancers, which are nothing more than chemical additives to trick your palate into thinking that it is a great product. Many of these additives, by the way, are the same chemicals given to laboratory rats to induce obesity so that weight-loss drugs may be developed.

There are a few exceptions. Some foods—seafood, fruit, and vegetables, for example—are quick-frozen just after picking.

Usually these products don't have any added ingredients, or at least no more than one. Quick-frozen shrimp or berries are easy to store and ensure that you always have some nutritious and flavorful food readily available. Healthy and nutritious olive oil is obviously in a package: a bottle. A bag of rice that is nothing but rice probably qualifies as real food. Bottom line, if you look at the ingredients, you will see that there is only one ingredient listed. This also qualifies as a real food.

However, select foods straight from the fresh-produce section, the fresh-meat section, and fresh nuts whenever possible. To go even further, try to choose organic products whenever selection and budget allow. While this does not completely guarantee that no chemicals have reached the food, it does go a long way toward providing a modicum of confidence that the food is real.

Another option is to buy locally grown produce or locally raised animal products. Many believe that this option is almost as good as organic. The theory is that local farmers are small farmers who take pride in the quality and safety of their products. In general, they use more conservative methods of treating insects on crops and illnesses that may occur in their animals. Plus, buying local usually means that products get to your table much quicker after harvest because they do not have to travel three thousand miles. This means that there is less opportunity for valuable minerals and vitamins to escape. And fresh produce or fish certainly has more flavor and tastes better than the same products that have been in shipment for five days.

If you really *do* need to purchase a food that is packaged, say a carton of skim milk, look carefully at all the ingredients. If an ingredient looks like a fake product, it probably is. If there are several suspicious ingredients, put it back on the shelf. A usual rule of thumb is: do not buy anything with more than three ingredients listed on the label. While one of these ingredients may, indeed, be chemicals, you are still a lot safer than choosing a product that has ten chemicals.

DIANE'S STORY

Unlike most of her friends, Diane always had a little weight problem. She called it *little* because she was usually somewhere between five to eight pounds overweight for her age and height, according to the doctors her mother took her to. In that time, not much was made of weight. "A healthy child" is what she was always called. But it didn't end there.

In college, she started gaining weight and just attributed it to the freshman spread. Then after she got married, she gained more. She justified that gain with the idea that you eat more when you're in love. But by the time she had her first child, she was about fifty pounds overweight, and had a serious talk with herself. She wasn't the cute, healthy child anymore; She was overweight and almost obese.

When she came to see me I recorded an inventory of foods that she was currently eating and encouraged her to start a food log. Gradually she began to see that the kind of food she was eating was contributing to her excess weight. She was preparing food the way her mother did: everything from a package! She even ate all of her fruits and vegetables from a package. It was easier to open a can of pears than to eat fresh ones. She realized that all of the preservatives and additives in the packaged foods were making her hungrier and not even giving her body the nutrients that it needed.

She lost fifty-five pounds over four months, and has kept it off for five years. Her new motto is "eat fresh, real food." Now, she makes everything from scratch, even soup. Once she learned to be organized and educated herself on how to cook, she couldn't believe how easy it was. She now truly believes that giving up processed food has been the main reason that she has maintained her ideal weight with very little effort.

KEY THREE: NO ARTIFICIAL SWEETENERS

One of the biggest hoaxes on the public has been the advent of artificial sweeteners. Early on, they were touted as a great way to enjoy your favorite sweet product without the dangers associated with eating and drinking lots of real sugar. They were certainly safe, since the FDA said so, and they did not spike the blood glucose like a real sugar product because the manufacturer said so. I think you probably know my opinion about this by now. Do not blindly trust what *they* tell you. Do your own research. Read small articles and studies, and see if they agree.

Recent university-based studies have shown that artificial sweeteners spike blood glucose just the same as a regular sugar product. Other studies have shown that people who drink diet soda weigh more than folks who drink real soda with sugar. How can that be? While there are the usual explanations about eating more because you think you are saving calories with your diet drink, I have a different theory. There are many who believe that your brain interprets artificial sugar in the same way it interprets real sugar, and I also think that this is true. This interpretation by the brain, that you are actually eating sugar, will cause a glucose spike in the same way that eating real sugar does. Whatever the cause of your blood-glucose spike, when it goes up, so do insulin levels, and your body proceeds to store fat. (This is the condensed version, by the way. The functions that cause this to happen require more of an explanation than is reasonable in this book.)

In my practice, I have had many people who choose diet drinks as their main beverage. They have anywhere from four to ten cans of diet soda a day. My experience has been that, unless these people give up this habit and begin drinking other liquids, they will not lose weight. If they manage to change their habits while on a weight-loss program, they almost always gain the weight back when they return to their old habit of drinking beverages with artificial sweeteners.

I hate to be the bearer of really bad news, but, folks, you will NOT keep your weight off if you don't give up, or at least cut down on, diet soft drinks, diet bottled teas, and diet powdered drinks. Any label that says diet or no calories is suspect. See if any artificial sweeteners are listed, and choose accordingly.

Most people consume the artificial sweeteners through beverages. Now you know that better, healthier choices exist. They just sound kind of boring. They don't have to be. Here are some easy, useful ideas to help kick the artificial-sweetener habit.

WATER

You know that drinking water is good for you, but, boy, that really doesn't sound interesting. Try giving it a flavor instead.

Squeeze fresh lemon or lime into your water. (This should be real lemon or lime that you actually cut and squeeze, not something poured out of a bottle.)

Try flavored waters, but look closely at the ingredients. Many will say zero calories but contain artificial sweeteners. Look for the ones that have flavors infused but nothing else added.

Or try making your own infused water. Add your own mint, basil, or other herbs and let it chill in the refrigerator. This choice makes a really refreshing drink, especially when it's hot or during a workout.

Add fresh fruit and let the water chill. This is refreshing and may actually add a bit of sweet flavor if you're really missing that taste. Oranges and strawberries are very good for this.

The best way to prepare this is to use a large glass pitcher and fill it with filtered water. If using oranges, for instance, peel the orange and use two or three slices. Prick each slice with a fork and drop all the slices into the water before chilling it. Do the same with strawberries or pineapple. I don't recommend putting just the juice in. The infused flavor is really what we're after.

OTHER BEVERAGES

Tea is a great beverage. It's healthy and flavorful and can be a good alternative to water if not brewed too strong. Of course, many of us were raised on sweet tea, and we find it's a habit that's really hard to break. I'm from the South, and I really had to work hard to give up my iced sweet tea, like Mama made, and start drinking unsweetened tea instead. I finally broke the habit by drinking other teas, not just black. When I switched to green tea, for example, I found that it was better without a sweetener. My taste buds adapted to the change, and gradually I preferred the unsweetened version. I no longer craved that sweet taste. Then I began to experiment with other flavors. I added lemongrass to the pot while it was brewing. I started making white tea, which is very delicate, and added my own fruit, just like previously suggested with water. I put blueberries and one drop of vanilla into the pot while it was brewing. This gave a lot of flavor to the tea and made it really tasty without using a sweetener.

Coffee is another beneficial beverage. It is, after all, from a berry with some of the same benefits as other berries. It's also somewhat of an appetite suppressant. The benefits are present, even in decaffeinated coffee. For this reason, many of my clients drink a small amount of coffee in the afternoon—about the time they get those late-in-the-day munchies. Research also shows that coffee inhibits the glucose spikes that lead to weight gain.

What you add to your coffee is another matter. Lots of cream and sugar are not great. Powdered and/or flavored creamers are just a bunch of chemicals, and you know how I feel about that. One or two ounces of fat-free milk is just fine. I'm not a big fan of adding sugar or artificial sweeteners to anything, including coffee. If you must have a sweet taste to the coffee, then half a package of Splenda or half a teaspoon of real sugar or honey is the least offensive. While I also like stevia as a product, many people cannot get past the bitter aftertaste. I usually limit patients to one package of Splenda per day.

JASON'S STORY

Jason is a sixty-five-year-old male who came to my office to lose about thirty-five pounds. He didn't want to come, but his wife insisted. He had numerous health problems, not the least of which was diabetes. He was on insulin but having very little success controlling his blood sugars. In fact, his fasting morning blood sugars were raging well into the 350 to 400 levels. (Normal is less than one hundred.) After taking a complete history, which included his daily food intake, I discovered that Jason's drink of choice was diet soda—he drank *five* liters a day. He loved the taste and the caffeine high. After all, there was no sugar in it, so he could drink at much as he wanted.

After discussing my concerns about the excessive artificial sweetener that he was ingesting, I suggested that he cut down to drinking no more than eight ounces a day. He resisted and complained. He really didn't believe me but agreed to try. Because he is an all-or-nothing kind of guy, he decided to stop, cold turkey. He went from drinking five liters a day to drinking zero.

When he came in one week later for a follow-up visit, he was beaming. His blood sugars had dropped from their highs of 400 to 125! Almost normal. He had to dramatically cut back his insulin levels, and his doctor was over the moon with delight.

"I never would have believed it if it hadn't happened to me," he said. "Thank you for this valuable insight that just may have helped save my life!"

OTHER FOODS

Our ancestors did not have very many sweet foods in their diet. Scientists have shown that they mostly ate protein, wild grasses, nuts, berries, and some occasional sweet fruits or honey. Of course, the sweet foods were a real treat. People looked forward to finding a sweet fruit and experiencing the pleasurable taste and feeling that comes from finding and experiencing these types of food. However, these foods were rare. They did not have a sweet treat once a day, much less several times a day. Again, if we follow the thinking that we are actually still very close to having the same genetic makeup as our ancestors, we would have to conclude that our bodies are not engineered for sweet or starchy foods (i.e., foods that increase your blood sugar) because they did not exist to any extent in the world of our ancient relatives.

My advice to my patients and clients is to minimize any baked desserts and pastries and ice creams. All of these foods have sugar or an artificial sweetener added to them. No matter which one is added, they both spike your blood sugar. While I don't believe in completely cutting out any food, I strongly suggest that these types of food be used as an occasional treat. In this case, I define occasional as no more than twice a month.

KEY FOUR: NO STARCHES

When I was growing up, we didn't use terms like "high glycemic" or "simple versus complex carbohydrates." We had carbohydrates, which referred to most vegetables, some fruits, and starches, which meant bread, pasta, potatoes, beans, except for green beans, all varieties of peas, rice, desserts, and really sweet fruits, like bananas. I find that, for most people, this is still the easiest way of explaining which carbs should be minimized in the diet.

When people come into my office and tell me they cut out carbs, they're usually referring to the agendas of other weight-loss programs that cut out everything but protein. This is not my belief. We are programmed to eat greens, salads, nuts, berries, and other basic, non-sweet fruits, like apples and pears. However, our bodies are not set up to have a constant exposure to anything that raises our blood sugar on a regular basis. This includes starches.

The word "starches" often refers to the white stuff. We all know it. Beans, corn, wheat products, and other grains also fall into this starchy category. A diet high in starchy carbohydrates, even healthy ones, is one of the most common causes of weight gain. Why?

Well, for starters, our bodies are not set up to handle all of the sugar that comes from eating a lot of these foods. Eating them sets up a cycle of increased blood sugar, increased insulin, and, finally, stored fat. If you eat a baked potato once a month, it's no big deal. If you eat cereal for breakfast, a baked potato for lunch, pasta with bread for dinner, and you do this three or four days a week, you have set up an environment where weight gain may occur. And remember, we're only talking about weight as measured on the scale. We're not even talking about increased risk of diabetes, high blood pressure, and heart disease.

And if you eat the unhealthy starches (you know, the potato chips, corn chips, snack crackers, and so on), then you have an even greater chance of adding up the pounds.

So why do we eat these things if they're bad for us and our bodies don't use them to our greatest health? Simply, because they make us feel good. They work on our brain and contribute to a release of endorphins, which gives us pleasure, even if only for a short time. But just like a drug addict, we start to really like that feeling, and so we eat more. And as we get used to that feeling and desire that feeling all the time, we eat more and more of the products that make us feel good. We all know the term "comfort food," don't we?

As more and more time goes by, we need more and more of these feel-good foods—pasta, mashed potatoes, bread, chocolate—to get the same high feeling. But as we pursue our high, we're also laying the groundwork to store fat. We are taking in so many products that literally turn directly into sugar that our bodies are overwhelmed with all this extra energy that we're not using. Unless you're training for the iron-man competition, you're not using the calories you take in. So, it gets turned into fat.

Most of you will not like this, but, TO KEEP WEIGHT OFF PERMANENTLY (and decrease all related health risks), YOU MUST DROP STARCHY FOODS FROM YOUR REGULAR DIET. Sorry, but it's the truth. Our bodies do *not* need these foods. But we were raised on them, and we like them.

I advise my clients to select their favorite food and figure out a way to add it in as a treat. For example, let's say there is a wonderful Italian restaurant in your town, and for years you and your spouse have gone there every Friday night. When you eat there, you usually have a glass of wine and bread while waiting to order. Then you have salad with bread and olive oil to start. Then you have pasta and, perhaps, one additional piece of bread. You enjoy another glass of Chianti. Then you split tiramisu with your spouse. If you look at this meal, you'll see that the major food group represented is carbohydrates, and starchy carbs at that. And where is the protein? What do you think this does to your blood sugar and your possibility of storing all of these calories as fat? Well, I'd say you have about a 99 percent chance that you have added to your stubborn, stored fat.

I'm a believer in adapting to your lifestyle. Your weekly outing to this restaurant with your spouse is important, and you have no intention of giving it up. I agree. But it's possible to make better choices. What's your favorite item in the above example? Well, if it's the pasta, then let's see how you can order differently. First, have the wine, but skip the bread. If your spouse really wants it, then ask the waiter to bring one or two slices but no more. Then how about having veal piccata (un-breaded) and a small side of pasta? Have double the salad and skip the extra bread. Have the wine, but skip the dessert. Have a coffee, regular or decaf, instead. Even though your pasta portion was smaller, you still enjoyed the taste of it and balanced out your meal better.

If you tell me that your favorite item is the bread, then limit to two pieces and don't have them until your salad comes. Then order your protein (veal, chicken, fish) with veggies or another salad or have your main meal be a large salad with chicken or fish. Have the wine and then coffee for dessert. I will give other examples later in this book, but I really want to emphasize that it's entirely possible to eat out, enjoy good food, and not gain weight.

Foods to cut out or eat as occasional treats include:

- ✧ White potatoes
- ✧ Sweet potatoes
- ✧ Pasta
- ✧ Bread
- ✧ Rice (brown and white)
- ✧ Yucca/taro
- ✧ Pastries
- ✧ Wheat products of any kind
- ✧ Dried fruits
- ✧ Sweet fruits (bananas, pineapples, melons, etc.)
- ✧ All grains
- ✧ All cereals
- ✧ Beans and peas (except for green beans)
- ✧ Corn products

Foods to eat often are:

- ✧ *Any* green, leafy vegetable
- ✧ Peppers
- ✧ Mushrooms
- ✧ Broccoli
- ✧ Cauliflower
- ✧ Asparagus
- ✧ Carrots

- ✧ Cucumbers
- ✧ Celery
- ✧ Fennel
- ✧ Tomatoes
- ✧ Brussels sprouts
- ✧ Artichokes
- ✧ Cabbage
- ✧ Summer squash
- ✧ Zucchini
- ✧ Onions
- ✧ Apples
- ✧ Pears
- ✧ Peaches
- ✧ All berries
- ✧ Avocado
- ✧ Plums
- ✧ Nectarines
- ✧ Cherries
- ✧ Grapes
- ✧ All citrus fruits

All vegetables and fruit should ideally be organic. As a reminder, it's always important to wash vegetables thoroughly, even organic vegetables. I use a product called Veggie Wash that uses natural citrus acids to remove the residues from all fruits and vegetables.

Also, fruits and vegetables should always be fresh or quick-frozen without any additional ingredients. Canned and dried are not ideal and should only be eaten sparingly.

It's important to have a balance between vegetables and fruits. Eating a whole pineapple, a cluster of grapes, two oranges, two apples, and one serving of broccoli a day is not good for your blood sugar either. Use common sense. Try to have a minimum of two vegetables for every one fruit per day.

A WORD ABOUT WHEAT

Of all the starchy, grain, and cereal products available, the worst, by far, are products made of wheat. When you eat pasta or bread, you are not eating products made from your grandparent's wheat. You're eating a highly modified product that has nothing to do with the wheat that our ancestors ate. In his book *The Wheat Belly*, Dr. William Davis gives you the total picture of why wheat is so horribly bad for you. I myself happen to be gluten intolerant and have not knowingly had any wheat product for many years now. All of my digestive symptoms—stomach aches, bloating, and IBS—have disappeared. But if I eat anything that contains wheat, say a salad dressing that has a wheat product used as a thickener, I immediately have stomach cramps and don't feel well.

But gluten intolerance is only one problem with wheat. In his book, Dr. Davis describes all of the other problems and really emphasizes how wheat spikes the blood sugar worse than almost every other product out there, including real sugar. If you take the time to read his book, I promise you will think long and hard before you ever put another wheat product into your mouth.

Now I know you folks from Italian decent are not happy with this advice. After all, Italians eat pasta. But, guys, you are not eating pasta made with wheat from the old country. Since wheat from the new country is not good for you, what can you do instead? I suggest looking for gluten-free pasta. I also suggest that you only use this as an occasional meal since rice pasta is still a starchy food that will spike blood glucose and lay down fat.

ANGIE'S STORY

Angie came to me to lose some weight. She needed to lose about thirty pounds, and because she was from a large Italian family, she was really having trouble cutting out pasta and bread. However, during the program she cut out all wheat products, as well as all other white products, and she lost about thirty pounds in ten weeks. I reviewed with her, in detail, exactly what she should do to keep the weight off. About six months later, she came back in to see me, and she had gained the weight back. She was angry and told me that my diet didn't work. When I asked her what she was doing differently, she said she had added back pasta, four or five times a week. She was very angry that she could not eat food that she felt was in her genetic makeup to eat without gaining weight. It was her God-given right, in fact, her duty, to eat pasta and bread like all good Italians. However, she once again cut out all wheat, lost the weight, and this time, she only added back a meal of gluten-free pasta once a week. I ran into her about two years later, and she had kept the weight off, lost another five pounds, and had maintained that weight for a year and a half. She became a believer.

OTHER STARCHY FOODS

Certain vegetables are also very starchy and will spike the blood glucose levels very quickly after being consumed. Root vegetables should always be eaten in moderation. Winter squash, beans, peas, and other starchy legumes should also be limited. If you're actually trying to lose weight, not just maintain, I would avoid all of these products until you reach your ideal weight, then add them back at the rate of one a week.

KEY FIVE: EAT YOUR (GOOD) FATS

When the low-fat, high-carb diet became popular in the United States, the health of Americans took a serious nose-dive. This was, and still is, a very unhealthy eating style, and one that is still being talked about, taught, and used. We really had it shoved down our throats that taking all fats out of our diets and eating fake fats instead was healthy. We were told that taking all dairy and animal fats out would reverse any trends toward increased heart disease. We replaced these fats with fake butter, omega-6 vegetable oils, trans fats, and other artery-clogging products. The trend for heart disease, diabetes, cancer, and other diseases did not go down but, instead, skyrocketed. Maybe somebody got it wrong.

There are a lot of helpful books and reports on the different kinds of fats and which are good and which are not. Since the purpose of this book is to give guidance and not quote scientific studies, I will not bore you with in-depth details about omega-6 versus omega-3 or olive oil versus corn oil. Rather, I choose to focus on the positive oils and fats and disregard the others (sort of).

Some of these fine scientific studies have shown that our problems with weight, heart disease, diabetes, and even cancers started when we adapted to a low-fat, high-carb way of eating. They have also shown that cultures eating high fats and minimal starchy carbs are much healthier than us Western folks. I have touched on this a bit already. As I said in chapter one, animals that are grass/pasture-fed do not have the same type of high saturated fat that animals have when they are raised in lots and forced to eat grains that are not part of their natural diet. This is one of the reasons that the French, who eat large amounts of beef and animal/dairy fat (like butter), have a lower incidence of heart disease and stroke. In the Mediterranean areas of Spain, France, Italy, and Greece, large amounts of olive oil are used. Although some residents of these regions are overweight, those who eat lots of olives, olive oil, avocados, and nuts are more likely to be at their ideal weight. This is especially true if they limit their starches, such as pasta. In the south of France, for example, they eat lots of olives, tapenade, goat cheese, foie gras, and lamb and are still much thinner than we are here in the United States.

Ideally, oils should be organic and minimally processed. Look for the words "cold pressed" and "expeller pressed" on the labels. I also look for "extra virgin" when I buy olive oil. If you use a product frequently, like olive oil, you can leave a small quantity out where it is handy. Otherwise, store oils in the refrigerator after opening.

My own experience has been that patients who eat some healthy fats every day and limit the unhealthy fats keep their weight off much easier than patients who cut out or minimize their fat intake.

Here are my lists of good fats and those to avoid.

GOOD FATS

Olive oil: use this as your main oil in dressings, marinades, and for some lower-heat cooking. You should be using more of this oil than any other.

Nut oils: I don't really use these myself, but some folks enjoy the different flavor for salads.

Salmon: wild salmon is best, as fish or game from the wild is leaner. Wild salmon is a great source of omega-3 and can be eaten a couple of times a week.

Walnuts: try to have ten or so as a snack or chop them up and add them to a salad.

Avocados: another good fat. I try to have at least one a week.

Coconut oil: there have been numerous claims made in recent years about the health and healing benefits of coconut oil. While I'm not sure if these benefits are true, I myself do use coconut oil at times, usually as a butter substitute. I often like the taste, and it seems a bit less oily in baked goods than large amounts of butter.

BAD FATS

The only *really* bad fats are what we call trans fats. Trans fats are artificially made when liquid fats are converted to a solid or semisolid state. They are, hands down, the absolute worse fat, and, please, eliminate *all* of them from your diet.

Examples of trans fats are commercially baked goods, like chips, pastries, snack crackers, and cookies; all other packaged snack foods (including microwavable popcorn); margarine; vegetable shortening; prepared icings; and candy bars.

In recent years, there has been so much negative publicity about trans fats that many food manufacturers and even fast-food chains are taking great pains to eliminate them from their products.

FATS TO USE IN MODERATION

Everything else; I don't see any reason to completely erase any type of fat *except* trans fats. Trans fats should be COMPLETELY erased from your diet. Period.

Perhaps this is a good time to define moderation. Experience with my patients has taught me that we all have our own ideas about how much actually defines a little or a lot. My definition of the word moderation is "no more than once a week and no more than two tablespoons." A small amount of organic butter on your asparagus is totally OK. A stick of butter is not. Use your common sense.

A TIDBIT

Do not choose foods that have large amounts of starch and fat. Use half a cup of olive oil a day if you want, just don't use all of it with pasta or bread. The combination of fat and starch seems to create a synergy between the two and will add pounds so fast that you won't believe it. Use your olive oil with veggies, salads, and in meat marinades. Use your pasta as a treat.

My definition of a treat is no more than twice a month.

MARY'S STORY

Mary is a software designer who was a victim of the low-fat diet theory. When she came in to see me to lose weight, she was well entrenched into the fat-is-bad mind-set. She ate no cheese, beef, or avocados. She used no oils, not even olive oil. Everything was nonfat. She ate egg whites only, mild white fish, and chicken breast. Because her food seemed tasteless, she relied heavily on packaged, processed nonfat foods and condiments. She was sixty pounds overweight, despite never eating any fat.

Mary was born in the sixties and grew up during the nonfat diet era. This is the way her mother ate and cooked. In college, all the girls ate this way. But it wasn't working for her.

I immediately suggested that Mary reverse course. I strongly suggested that she start eating whole eggs, small bits of cheese, avocados, salmon, and real salad dressing with olive oil. While most of us eat these items without any thought, Mary practically had a panic attack when I strongly urged her to change her diet in this small way. It took a couple of weeks for her to get the courage to change, but she was feeling desperate, and her way just wasn't working. So she made these changes, and, after one week, she came back to see me. While she had lost three and a half pounds, it was her attitude and energy that were so thrilling. She *felt* so much better. She wasn't hungry, and her food actually had some taste to it even though she had given up the fake chemical enhancers she had been using.

She became much more open to change after that, and I'm pleased to report that she lost sixty-two pounds and has kept it off for over three years. She called me recently to say she was moving and thanked me for all of the help I had given her. She told me that, in addition to the changes I helped her make, she has added coconut oil, flax oil, and additional wild salmon to her diet on a regular basis. She knows the difference between good fats and trans fats and never worries about the good fats. She feels satisfied with her food now, and she owes it all to fat.

KEY SIX: WATCH THE SCALE

There's a saying that "you can't change what you can't measure." I find that to be absolutely true. When patients come back to see me after they've lost their original weight and then gained some back, half of them have stopped weighing themselves every morning. They decided that as long as they could fit into their clothes, they were OK.

Now, ladies, you all know that we can gain weight just by thinking about ice cream. (At least it feels like it!) My patients all reported that they had gained anywhere from eight to twenty-five pounds before they knew it. These are the folks who had stopped weighing themselves and just went by the feel of their waistbands.

Here's what seems to happen. Let's say someone loses twenty-five pounds. They quit weighing themselves and also start eating a few more starches again. Before they know it, they've gained back five pounds. "Not so bad," they say to themselves, "because I'm still down twenty pounds." What they don't stop to realize is that five pounds represents 20 percent of what they originally lost. That's a lot. A 20 percent gain is really a lot. It sets up a situation where the body is comfortable putting weight back on, and it changes the momentum of the body from stabilizing to gaining.

My advice is to establish a routine for your daily weigh-in: roll out of bed, urinate, weigh yourself, and write it down.

Yes, I know we all travel and that there are times we don't have access to a scale. Do the best you can. Most hotels and, certainly, cruise ships have spas or workout facilities, and most of these facilities have scales. Try to weigh at the same time and under the same conditions every morning when away from your normal scale. For example, if you're on a cruise, try to go at the same time, say, eight o'clock in the morning, with the same type of clothes say light gym shorts, T-shirt and shoes every morning. You'll be able to establish a base when you first arrive, and you will at least be able to see if you're maintaining or gaining.

JACK'S STORY

Jack came to see me six years ago because he felt that he needed to lose about twenty-five pounds. His clothes were getting too tight, and he didn't want to buy more. Because Jack is a high-profile professional who is often seen around town, it was very important for him to make a good impression on people. He wore expensive clothes and wanted to make sure he looked great in them.

Jack lost thirty-three pounds and kept it off for several years. However, the hectic schedule of business lunches and evening dinner meetings started taking its toll. Four years after he first lost the weight, he came back into my office for help. His clothes were suddenly tight again, and he felt fat.

When I got Jack on the scale, he had gained twenty-three pounds without even knowing it. Although I had counseled Jack on the importance of weighing regularly, he tended to ignore my advice. He was busy, and weighing every morning was something people who were obsessed with their weight did. He figured that if his clothes started getting too tight it meant that he had put on two or three pounds, and he would just watch his diet for a couple of days and take it off. He was shocked when he saw the number on the scale.

Jack lost the weight again, and this time he incorporated some additional habits into his routine, the first one being to weigh himself every morning. When I ran into him two years later, he looked great and had not gained a single pound. He saw the wisdom of the saying that "you can't change what you do not measure."

KEY SEVEN: PROTEIN DAYS

This is going to be your secret weapon. Here it is: *if you gain more than two pounds, do a protein day.*

This is the secret I use to help people keep the weight off for good. I personally do not know of one former patient who has gained the weight back while following this advice. The simple reason why this works is that when your ratio of protein to carbohydrates gets out of balance—with your intake of carbs being a lot greater than your intake of lean protein— you will hold on to water before you start actually accumulating fat. When you see the scale go up two pounds or more, then you're actually getting a heads-up that true weight gain is just around the corner. By doing a protein day, you bring your body back into balance, and you will release the water, usually through the kidneys, over the next day or two. Then, if you go back to the other principles outlined in this book, you will continue to maintain your weight.

Caution: I advise you to never do more than one protein day at a time. Also, *this is not a crutch.* If you think you can just eat anything you want and do a protein day twice a week, your body will get wise, and this trick will quit working. The body is pretty smart that way.

So what does a protein day consist of? It's very simple and easy. The entire day's food intake consists of protein, except for the evening meal, when a small salad or piece of fruit is allowed. That's it. Any type of protein will do.

Here is an example of a protein day:

- Have two hard-boiled eggs with a quarter cup of non-fat cottage cheese for breakfast.
- Have one large chicken breast or a quarter to half a pound of steamed shrimp (with more nonfat cottage cheese if you like) for lunch.
- For dinner, have six to eight ounces of steak or fish, a small salad with romaine lettuce, and one tablespoon of olive-oil dressing (you can make it yourself or, if in a hurry, use Newman's Own).
- Snacks should also be protein. Extra chicken, shrimp, or boiled eggs works really well.

The next day, return to your normal, healthy eating plan described earlier in this book. That is, eating between 25 to 40 percent of your daily food intake in lean protein and the remainder in vegetables, low-glycemic fruits, and small amounts of good fat or foods that contain good fats, like walnuts and avocados.

I have very rarely had a case where this does not work. You may not see the results the next day, but you will the day after. This is usually the case with myself. It seems that if I am bad on Monday, I don't see a weight gain until Wednesday. Likewise, if I have a protein day on Wednesday, I usually don't see my weight return to its previous number until Friday.

Most patients find this extremely easy to do. They usually report that they feel really good on the protein day. Also, most of them report that, after a protein day, they tend to urinate more for the next eight to twelve hours, so be aware that you may wake up during the night for a bathroom visit.

I want to again emphasize that THIS IS NOT A CRUTCH. The body, especially the female body, has a tendency to be a bit too smart for its own good sometimes. It starts to recognize patterns, and when you overuse a trick, such as the protein day, it will get wise and quit responding. It's as though it's saying, "Hey, I know what you're doing, and I don't want to play ball anymore. I'm going to stay at this weight." Also, doing more than one protein day in a row is *not* something I advocate. Eating ONLY protein for several days in a row is not a nutritionally or metabolically sound plan. If you abuse the protein day, then over time you will not be taking in enough quality nutrients that are required for good health.

It's important that you follow the two-pound rule in order to keep your weight stable. Following this rule requires that you know your weight set point. My definition of the weight set point is this: the weight that you are at the day you finish your program is your weight set point. If you have not done a formal program, then pick the weight that you feel the happiest at. If you lost twenty-two pounds and then gained two back the first week you strayed from your program but stayed at the new weight for two weeks, then your body has settled into that weight. That is your weight set point.

If you got on your scale this morning and are up two and a half pounds over your base weight set point, then you must take action today. Yes, I know you have lunch with your friends and a dinner party this evening, but you really do have to act today. Based on my years of experience with thousands of patients, this is an area where people can mess up. They decide that today will not be convenient, so they will have to wait a couple of days. In a couple of days, they are up another pound, and the body's momentum has now shifted to gaining weight. If this occurs, then doing a protein day does not result in the same benefits, and getting that three or four pounds back off is going to be a lot harder.

Patients who have kept their weight off and remain at a stable, healthy weight report that, after three to six months, they rarely need to do a protein day. Their bodies have adjusted to their new way of eating, and they have adopted the correct protein-to-carbohydrate ratio that works for them. They just seem to automatically eat the right things. However, most of them also report that doing the protein days occasionally during the first few months really seemed to help stabilize their weight faster. After six months, most patients report that their weight is stable without any protein days at all.

MARIA'S STORY

Maria is a beautiful Latino woman with silky long black hair and porcelain skin. She is tall and has a shape that most of us would do anything to have. When she came to my office, she had been living in the United States for about two years and found that she was gaining weight despite eating what she felt was a healthy diet. She wanted guidance to lose the weight and keep it off.

After completing a six-week diet program, we began to look at how she could maintain her weight. One of the tools that we used was the two-pound rule with the protein day. Maria completely embraced this concept, and I did not hear from her again.

Four years later, I ran into Maria on the street. She looked wonderful and had clearly kept the weight off. "Wow," I said. "Whatever you're doing is certainly working. You look very fit and fabulous."

She replied that she owed everything to that one little trick. "What trick?" I asked.

"The protein day," she said. "I only use it now and again, but, boy, does it work. My weight has stayed stable now for the entire four years, and I don't really have to work at it. Thank you so much for all of your help. I've learned to eat in my new country and not gain weight. It's great!"

KEY EIGHT: BE PREPARED

Let's be honest. We all have busy lives. In fact, most of us are more than busy. We're stressed, harried, overwhelmed, and constantly on the go. We have fifty things on our agenda today and only time to do eight. I know because I'm right there with you.

So, take a deep breath before you get mad that I'm going to add another item to your agenda, and let's talk this through. No matter what you do, no matter what your career and the demands that go with it, no matter if you are a stay-at-home mom, a soccer mom, a Red Cross volunteer, or a corporate executive, you will perform better if you're eating a nutritionally sound diet. Not only that, but no matter what method you used to lose weight, I'm sure you worked hard. You were proud when you lost weight and were able to wear your old clothes again. You owe it to yourself to honor that good effort and make a commitment to never go back to that situation again.

This is about taking care of you. You will be healthier, happier, and feel better overall if you're eating right. You will be better able to cope with your role as mother, attorney, salesman, or software designer. Unfortunately, it takes a bit of planning for that to happen. The right foods don't just magically appear in your refrigerator.

I don't know your life. Only you know the demands and frenzy that happens with your job or family. But there are a few points that can help everyone.

Spend one hour a week planning and shopping. You must have an agenda. Otherwise you will be at the mercy of your cravings or impulses when you get to the grocery store.

Review your schedule for the week. Do you eat out at lunch, or do you take your lunch? Do you have dinner with clients on Wednesday, or does the family all have a night out on Friday? Take this into consideration when making your grocery list.

Don't buy more food than you need for the week. This is a good rule to follow for at least a month or six weeks. If you decide to stock up on a food, you will see a lot of it when you open the refrigerator and be tempted to eat more. Let's say you take cottage cheese and an apple to work every day for a snack. Then buy five apples and one container of cottage cheese. This also helps prevent waste since you might be tired of apples next week.

Make a list of the restaurants where you know you can get good veggies and a lean protein, such as fish or chicken. I'm in a situation where I eat out a lot. Because of my schedule, I only cook on weekends, when I have more time. During the week, I usually eat dinner out at a restaurant. I've learned which ones are best suited to my way of eating. I know that most Italian restaurants don't work well for me because I don't eat pasta. However, there is one in my town that will prepare poached salmon and broccoli for me. I often add a Caesar salad, and I have a great meal. Since I live in Florida, there are a number of places where I can get good fish, fresh veggies, and a salad. However, it took quite some time for me to really get a working list of the restaurants that I know I can count on for the kind of foods I want. Start your list now.

Set aside some time once a week to prepare the foods you need to have on hand. If you take your lunch to work, then cook your chicken ahead of time, and keep it in the refrigerator. It will keep for a few days without any problems. Boil your eggs ahead of time. They also keep really well and are an easy food to grab quickly if you're in a hurry. Many of my patients have told me that the easiest thing for them to do is prepare their chosen food, say, chicken, and put it in individual bags or containers. Then they will add their apple, berries, or other fruit, and they find that their mornings are basically free of stress. All they have to do is grab their container and hustle the kids out the door for school.

Salad seems to be one of the items that can be difficult to prepare ahead. If you need to take a green salad made with lettuce or spinach, prepare it the night before, not two days before, and don't put the dressing on. You will need to take some dressing in a separate container to put on when you are ready to eat it. Likewise, if you eat tomatoes, slice them when you're ready to eat them.

If you take fruit as part of your meal or snack, decide if you want to eat it whole or sliced. Many of my patients like to take their apples or pears already peeled and sliced, but if you do that the night before, then they may turn brown. Avoiding this would require a little prep work in the morning. Analyze your schedule. If preparing food in the morning does not fit into your schedule, then don't put pressure on yourself. Make an easier choice.

Don't rule out your grocery store. Maybe you can count on having time to run out at lunch. Maybe it's easier for you to take a break and get food than it is for you to prepare food at home. If this describes you, then large grocery stores can be a lifesaver. Most will have premade salads, preboiled eggs, baked chicken breast, and other possible choices. I don't recommend deli meat products because of their high sodium content and additives, but other items provide quick, healthy choices.

Find a coach. If you're struggling with this aspect of your life, then try finding a good weight-loss/nutrition coach. A good coach will be able to assess your life and give you valuable guidance. A good coach will also encourage and assist you with problem solving if you're stuck and don't know how to organize your food or eating options. The feedback from my patients is that, of all the services I offer, this is the one that they really find invaluable. They tell me that this ability to help them solve food dilemmas is one of the most important parts, maybe the most important, of my program. If you decide to look for a coach, I would suggest that your first encounter with this coach be in the form of a conversation, whether in person or by phone. If you're comfortable with your choice, then, often, you can do future sessions by e-mail or Skype.

GINGER'S STORY

Several years ago Ginger had gained about twenty-five pounds and was miserable. She came to see me and participated in a ten-week weight loss program. She lost twenty-six pounds during that program and felt and looked great. Her energy level was the highest it had been in years. And, most importantly, she felt good about herself, and it showed at work when she met daily with clients.

Well, let's fast-forward four years. She was in the middle of a very stressful building project and had completely lost her way as far as her eating habits went. She had joined the grab-and-go set, and we all know what kinds of food are available to just grab. It came to a head when her husband caught her eating a Twinkie and insisted she stop and call me that very day.

She called and let me know that she needed immediate help. I saw her right away and let her know that she could get back on track with a little organization.

She lost the weight again, but, most importantly, I helped her set up a schedule and a way to plan her meals so that she was not hungry and could eat on the go if she needed to. We worked together to plan meals, snacks, and grocery lists. We organized a routine for food preparation at home. I encouraged her to take thirty minutes around midday to decompress, even if she didn't have time for a leisurely lunch.

Well, this turned out to be exactly the type of help she needed. She lost the weight, felt better, and had plenty of time and energy to finish her stressful project. "I encourage everyone to seek help if you feel overwhelmed with the idea of organizing your food," she later said. "With a few tips and the help of a good coach, it can be really easy. I know, because it worked for me."

LET'S REVIEW

Here's a quick review of everything that we've discussed. Use it as a quick reference if you find that you need to refresh your memory about the *Gone for Good!* basics.

Eat 25 to 40 percent of your food as lean protein. Most any animal protein source is OK. Limit processed, preserved, and canned meats to one serving a month. Protein sources should be organic, grass-fed, and hormone-free.

Small amounts of dairy are OK. Products should come from grass-fed, organically raised cows. Even so, use nonfat milk and yogurt when possible.

Eat real food. Reduce or eliminate canned products and foods with more than three ingredients. Get rid of processed, prepackaged foods. This one guideline will greatly reduce your exposure to chemicals. Eating real food also helps you to avoid developing food addictions caused by combinations of certain additives.

Eat organic as much as possible. This also helps reduce exposure to toxic, potentially harmful chemicals and their effects on our bodies.

Eliminate artificial sweeteners. All of them! If you need a little sweet taste in your coffee or tea, then one package of Splenda per day is acceptable. Stevia is also OK.

Eliminate starches, especially grains. Pasta, potatoes, and rice are not your friends. These are treat foods. Most people seem to be able to have one of these a week, but no more. This also assumes that you're not having a sugary, starchy dessert as well. Think about what you really miss, and figure out a way to have that food, but cut out other culprits. Balance is the key.

Eat good fats. Use olive oil, and eat walnuts and fatty fish, like wild salmon. Have a small amount of real butter or cream (organic). Low-fat diets have failed miserably. I don't limit all fats, just bad fats used in fried or snack foods.

Weigh yourself every morning. This allows you to know if you're staying on track.

Know your weight set point. This is the weight that you have stabilized at for two or three weeks or the weight that you were at when you finished your structured program. Weight set points can be revised downward, but not up.

Follow the two-pound rule. If you gain two or more pounds over your weight set point, then you must do a protein day. Refer back to Key Seven to get the details of how to do a protein day correctly.

Be prepared. This puts you in control of your food, not the other way around.

SAMPLE DAILY MENU

Breakfast: four ounces of nonfat cottage cheese, half a cup of blueberries, coffee with one ounce of nonfat milk

Snack (if needed): one apple (any size or variety), half an ounce of hard cheese, or half a boiled egg

Lunch: four or five ounces of grilled chicken, spinach salad with any kind of veggies (no croutons), and one tablespoon of salad dressing made with olive oil

Snack (if needed): ten to fifteen grapes or one ounce of left-over chicken

Dinner: four or five ounces of wild salmon (baked or grilled); steamed, mashed cauliflower with one teaspoon of olive oil, herbs, and half an ounce of grated Parmesan; a small green salad or zucchini sautéed in one tablespoon of olive oil with herbs as a second vegetable; and one glass of wine, preferably red

Dessert: decaf coffee or tea with nonfat milk or, if you really need something, half of an apple baked with cinnamon, nutmeg, or any other spice you wish

A WORD ABOUT EXERCISE

Our bodies need movement. They were built for activity and various types of motion. Our ancestors were constantly moving about just to secure the food needed for survival. But I have seen no evidence that our methods of working out two hours every day is helpful for weight loss or weight maintenance. It seems odd to me that we have to spend time *burning off* what we *take in*.

Observation of my patients has taught me that when you eat the correct food in the correct ratios for your lifestyle, you're not hungry and have enough energy for anything that you do. If you like to cycle every morning, then you will be able to adjust your food intake for your activity. This is also where a good coach can help.

Having said all of this, I myself try to have at least an hour of concentrated activity every day. This is far less than some advisors would suggest. But I find that my weight remains stable no matter which activity I choose, or even if I'm busy and skip a week. I choose to be active because I happen to like going to the gym. I think I have more energy when I vary my workouts between weights, cardio classes, and yoga. But I don't do these activities to burn calories. I do them because I feel good doing them.

ONE FINAL THING

Relax. This is not as hard as it may seem in the beginning. You will not starve. You will not be hungry, cranky, or wither away if you cut out bread. I promise. You will feel and look great. You will have lots of energy. And your health will improve.

Yes, this will take some thought and possible attitude adjustment. But I believe that most of you have been through things in your life that are much harder than sticking to this way of eating. In fact, most of my patients do not find this hard. While it may be challenging in the first two or three weeks, it will begin to become second nature after that.

I've listened to the stories of my patients, and I'm constantly amazed by the courage and dedication of people in general: the difficult fad diets, the three-hour workouts, the eating disorders, and the surgeries—all to achieve a look, a feeling, and overall health. If you have the drive and courage to do any (or all) of these things, you will be on easy street with this way of eating.

My goal in writing this book is to give all of you an easy, common-sense way to maintain your weight loss and maximize the health and self-esteem benefits that have come with that weight loss. My goal is to provide simple-to-understand directions to ensure that you will NEVER gain any of that weight back. EVER! My goal is that you will continue to be the best that you can be.

JIM'S STORY

When Jim and his wife Lena came to my office for a free consultation, it was perfectly clear that Jim did not want to be there. He didn't think he *needed* to be there. He was in total control of his life, and no one would tell him differently.

Jim was a big guy at six feet, three inches tall, but he really needed to lose thirty-five or forty pounds. He had high cholesterol, high blood pressure, and was borderline diabetic. He liked good food and drinks and really loved to go to fine restaurants. Jim's wife was clearly worried and did most of the talking. Jim was too sullen to say much. She explained that, at his age (fifty-six), he had several health issues that needed to be addressed. She loved him and wanted to keep him around. His kids loved him and wanted him to be around to see his grandkids. She admitted that she had practically dragged him to the consultation and that she would do whatever it would take to help him lose weight and decrease his cholesterol, blood pressure, and glucose levels.

I discussed the program, outlined what would happen during the ten weeks, and then I told them both that I would not be interested in accepting Jim as a patient unless he was totally on board. That statement made him perk up. I would refuse to accept his money if he did not buy into the program mentally and emotionally.

Well, the challenge was just too much for him to resist. So, his answer was yes! Lena broke into tears when Jim decided that he would try. He promised to really try. He prided himself on sticking to his commitments and coming out a winner.

And keep his commitment he did. He lost fifty pounds and was so shocked at how easy it was that I do believe I have a friend for life. He told everyone about me. He sent in friends as patients. He was as good as his word and kept his promise to his wife to keep it off for good.

You see, the last time I saw Jim and Lena, they had just come from their daughter's wedding. Jim had kept his weight off for about eight months by then, and I wondered how he had managed the wedding. It was a big affair with lots of before-wedding dinners and celebrations. He grinned. He had enjoyed himself very much. Yes, he did have some wedding cake. Yes, he did have some lasagna. Yes, he did have an extra glass of champagne. But he remembered the rules and kept his ratio of protein to carbohydrates in balance. He didn't gain any weight.

"This is the easiest thing I have ever done," he said as he gave me a big hug. "Thank you for giving me a new lease on life."

MY STORY

I offer free consultations for people who are thinking about starting a weight-loss program or hiring a weight-loss coach. One of the first questions I'm asked is, "Did you lose weight on this program?" or "How do you keep your weight off?" Because people are curious about the background of the person giving them advice, I'm happy and honored to share my story with you.

I graduated from nursing school with a bachelor's degree in nursing. During my four years of study, I only had one class on nutrition. Interestingly, since I was at a large medical university where many other modalities were being trained, that class also included the second-year medical students. This was the only nutrition class they received during their training as well.

The instructor was dry, uninspiring, and uninteresting. Everyone there hated the class. Except me. I loved it. I totally looked forward to that class, and I took on the challenge of inspiring myself to read the text and memorize the facts. I was the only student in that class to receive an A.

Since that time, I have worked in many areas of medicine. I have worked in critical-care units, surgery, been a leader in various areas of the hospitals, been a visiting home care nurse, and run private doctors' offices. And yet, all of my continuing education, as well as my outside consulting, has centered on nutrition and the role it takes in healing. I have taken many nutritional classes—some traditional, but most with a holistic theme. When I was diagnosed with breast cancer at the age of forty-two, I worked with a naturopath and nutritionist who specialized in cancer. This was in addition to working with regular oncologists.

But, believe it or not, one of my biggest challenges occurred when I went through menopause. I gained about thirty-five pounds while doing all of the things I thought were right. I did walking marathons, weight training three times a week, Pilates two times a week, and cycling once a week. I ate a 1,200-calorie diet with no alcohol.

And during part of this time, I gained about two pounds a week. And no, it was NOT muscle.

I was irritated. I think many of you can identify with that. I spent about a year or so doing research and came up with the wonderful weight-loss program that I use today with my clients.

But, that was not the end of the story. Yes, I lost the thirty pounds and then lost about five more and got to the weight that I was at in college. But, then what? How to keep it off?

There were no really firm guidelines out there—at least none that made sense to me. So I set out to develop my own. Again, I spent about a year reading, researching, and experimenting (on myself) to find the perfect combination that would allow a stable weight while being very easy to understand and incorporate into my daily life. The guidelines that I have shared with you in this book have come directly from my own research and from a deeper understanding of the roles of proteins, carbs, and fats. But mostly, they have also come from the stories and the anecdotal evidence of my patients. These patients have been, and continue to be, my greatest teachers.

FURTHER READING

Cordain, Loren. *The Paleo Diet.* Hoboken, NJ: John Wiley & Sons, Inc. 2011

Davis, William. *The Wheat Belly.* New York: Rodale, Inc. 2011

Kessler, David. *The End of Overeating.* New York: Rodale, Inc. 2009

Graham, Gray, Deborah Kesten, and Larry Scherwitz. *Pottenger's Prophecy—How Food Resets Genes for Wellness or Illness.* Amherst, MA: White River Press, 2011

Wolf, Robb. *The Paleo Solution.* Victory Belt Publishing 2010

ACKNOWLEDGEMENTS

I would like to thank a few people who have contributed to the production of *Gone for Good!* First, I would like to thank the staff at BodySculptingMD who have assisted our patients and have helped to make their weight loss and weight management experiences pleasurable. Particularly, Zsuzsanna, who seems to always have the right word of encouragement ready at a moment's notice.

Also, thanks to my friends who encouraged me to share my experiences and knowledge. Grace, Carla and Lynne, thank you for your kind words and support.

And finally, thanks to my husband, Mark Walter, MD, who used every opportunity to sing my praises and encouraged me to use my expertise to help others. Thank you, baby!

ABOUT THE AUTHOR

Susan Lewis, RN, BSN, graduated from the Medical University of South Carolina. She has worked as a nurse manager in hospitals, outpatient facilities, and private-practice facilities. Her true love and in-depth experience has been in the field of nutrition and nutritional counseling. She has worked with cancer patients, AIDS patients, and has coached clients in overall health practices. She is best known for her weight-loss and weight-management programs, which boast a 90 percent success rate. She is available for private consultations and group seminars. She may be reached at susanlewisrn@aol.com.

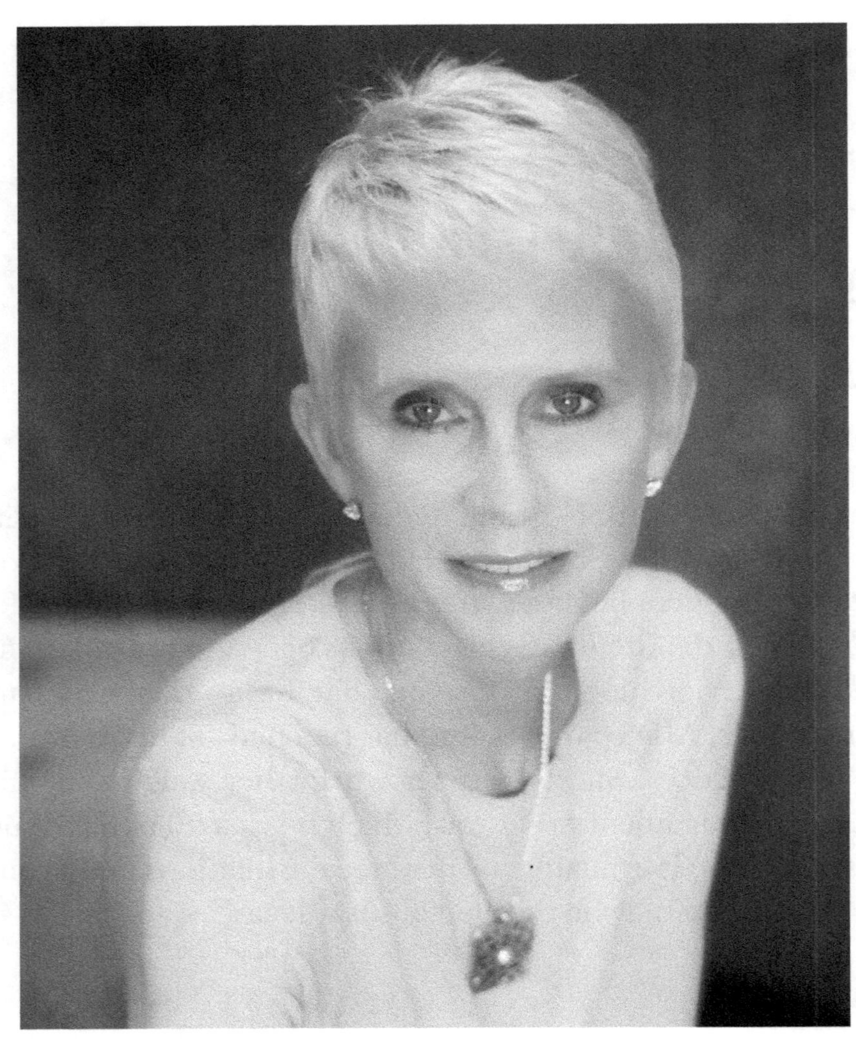